Up to A Weight Loss?

Try These 30 Detox Recipes to Get Rid of Harmful Toxins!

BY

Carla Hale

License Notes

No part of this Book can be reproduced in any form or by any means including print, electronic, scanning or photocopying unless prior permission is granted by the author.

All ideas, suggestions and guidelines mentioned here are written for informative purposes. While the author has taken every possible step to ensure accuracy, all readers are advised to follow information at their own risk. The author cannot be held responsible for personal and/or commercial damages in case of misinterpreting and misunderstanding any part of this Book

Table of Contents

Introduction

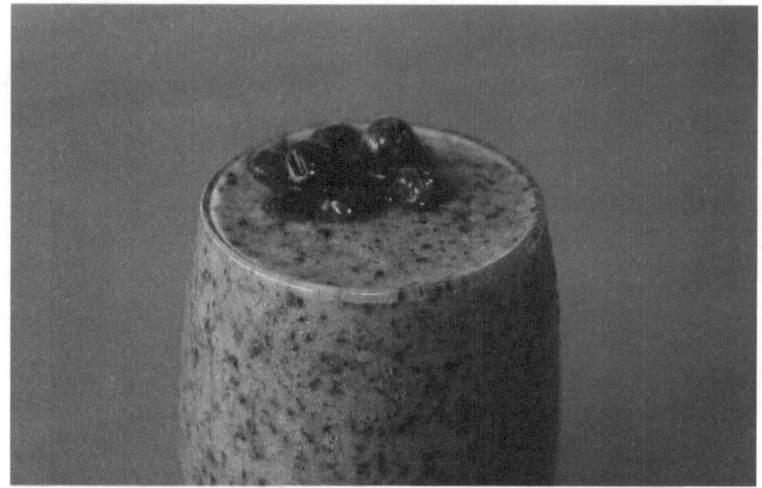

Detoxification and detox are also known as body cleansing and it aims to get rid of the harmful toxins which prevail in the body. Detox recipes aim to cleanse and purify the body off harmful substances and purifies it.

With the help of some foods, your body can get rid of these toxins such as foods that are rich in vitamins and iron. Some detox smoothies also serve this cause and they can make your immune system stronger, make you look young, keep your skin hydrated and speed up your metabolism.

It is important to maintain a healthy diet while taking in these juices just so as not to harden the process of keeping your body in a good state. It is advisable to cut down on your carb intake and increase your take in of proteins found in meat, fish, eggs; fruits, vegetables, whole grains etc.

Soups are a good food item to add to your healthy eating plan as they are light and quick to digest.

We trust that you will have a great read and jump up to a keeping your healthy as much as possible.

Remember to use fresh produce for these recipes as the fresh natural juices of the ingredients help in making the process more effective.

Kale and Apple Detox Smoothie

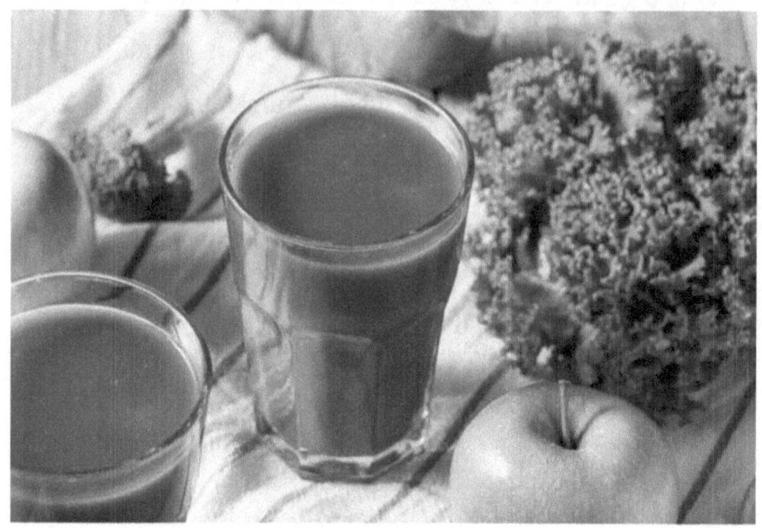

Description: Kale and apple both are very rich in iron and act as excellent antioxidants. They speed up the metabolism process and help in reducing weight. You should drink at least one glass a day of this kale and apple detox smoothie.

Preparation Time: 5 minutes.

Serves: 3.

Ingredients:

- Almond milk- 2/3 cup
- Ice- ¾ cup
- Chopped kale- 1 ½ cups
- Chopped celery- 1 stalk
- Red or green apple- ½
- Flax seeds- 1 tablespoons
- Honey-1 teaspoon

Directions:

1. Chop the kale.
2. Chop the celery.
3. Cut apple into small pieces.
4. Take a blender and add in the chopped kale, chopped celery, apple, ice, almond milk, honey and the flax seeds and blend so that all the ingredients are mixed properly.
5. Add more almond milk if it is required.
6. Pour into glasses and serve!

Detox Tea

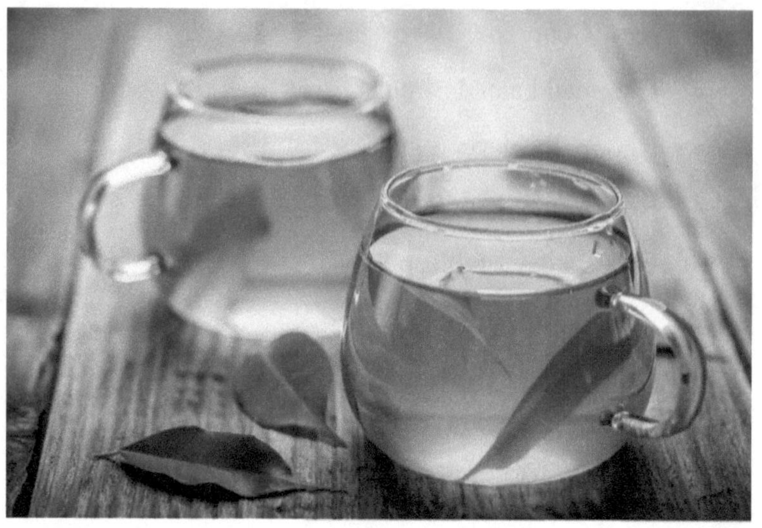

Description: Detox tea can benefit your immune system significantly.

Preparation Time: 5 minutes

Serves: 1

Ingredients:

- Warm water- 1 cup
- Apple cider vinegar- 2 tablespoons
- Lemon juice- 2 tablespoons
- Honey- 1 tablespoon
- Cinnamon- 1 teaspoon
- Cayenne- a pinch

Directions:

1. Take a cup, and add in the warm water, apple cider vinegar, lemon juice, honey, cinnamon and the cayenne and mix properly so that all the ingredients are mixed in properly.
2. Enjoy while your tea is warm!

Pineapple Banana Detox Smoothie

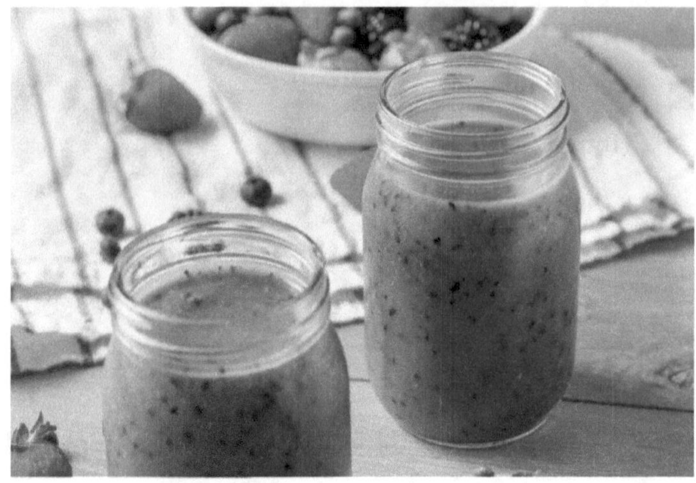

Description: This smoothie is made with a combination of pineapples and bananas. Bananas are great for our immune system and both the pineapple and the banana are great antioxidants and help a lot in reducing weight. This detox smoothie has some great health benefits for your body.

Preparation Time: 5 minutes.

Serves: 2.

Ingredients:

- Pineapple- 1
- Banana-1
- Apple- 1
- Spinach- 2 cups
- Water- 1 cup

Directions:

1. Cut the pineapple into chunks.
2. Cut the banana into slices.
3. Peel and core the apple.
4. Wash, dry and cut the spinach.
5. Take your blender and add in the pineapple, banana, apple, spinach and water and blend so that all the ingredients are mixed properly.
6. Add more water if the consistency of the smoothie is thick.
7. Pour into glasses and serve!

Kale, Pineapple and Coconut Detox Smoothie

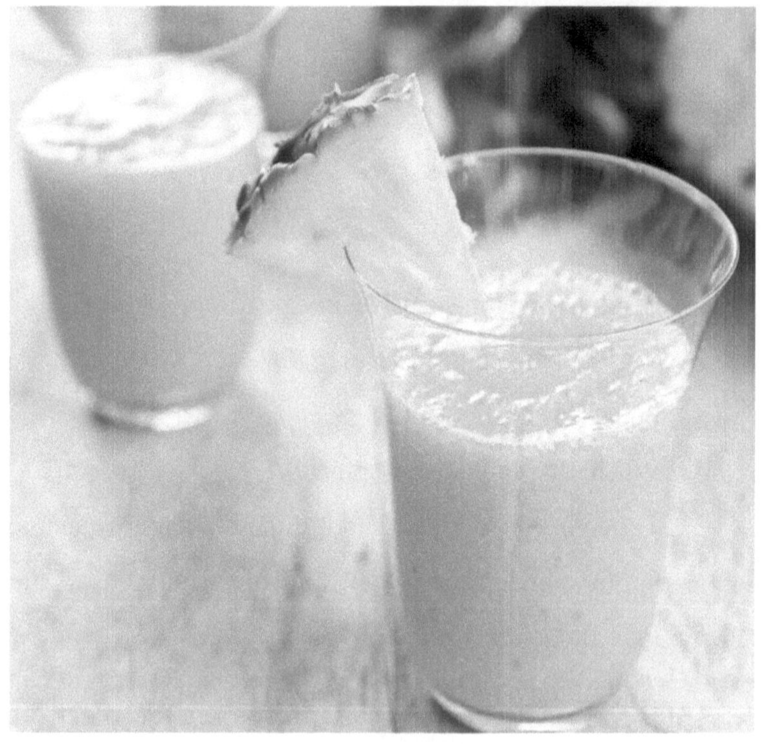

Description: This smoothie is made with the combination of kale, pineapple and coconut. All three of these contribute to a good health and help in reducing weight. They are loaded with iron and vitamin C and increase the rate of metabolism as well.

Preparation Time: 5 minutes.

Serves: 2.

Ingredients:

- Banana- 1
- Pineapple- 1
- Coconut water- 1 cup
- Chopped kale- 2 cups

Directions:

1. Cut the banana into small pieces.
2. Cut the pineapple into chunks
3. Cut and chop the kale.
4. Take your blender and add in the banana, pineapple, coconut water and the chopped kale and mix all the ingredients properly.
5. Pour into glasses and serve!

Avocado Detox Smoothie

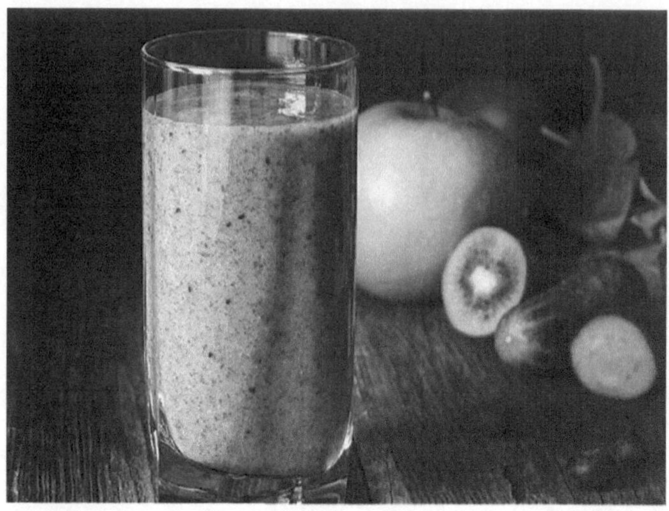

Description: Avocados are very good for our health. They help in keeping the cholesterol level in the body to a minimum and are great for our skin as well. This smoothie is full of iron because it includes apple and spinach as well.

Ingredients:

- Apple juice- 1 ½ cups
- Spinach or kale- 2 cups
- Apple- 1
- Avocado- ½

Directions:

1. Peel the apple and cut into slices.
2. Chop and cut the spinach or kale.
3. Cut and chop the avocado.
4. Take your nutribullet cup and add in the spinach, apple, avocado and the apple juice.
5. Mix together all the ingredients.
6. Pour into glasses and serve!

Apple Detox Smoothie

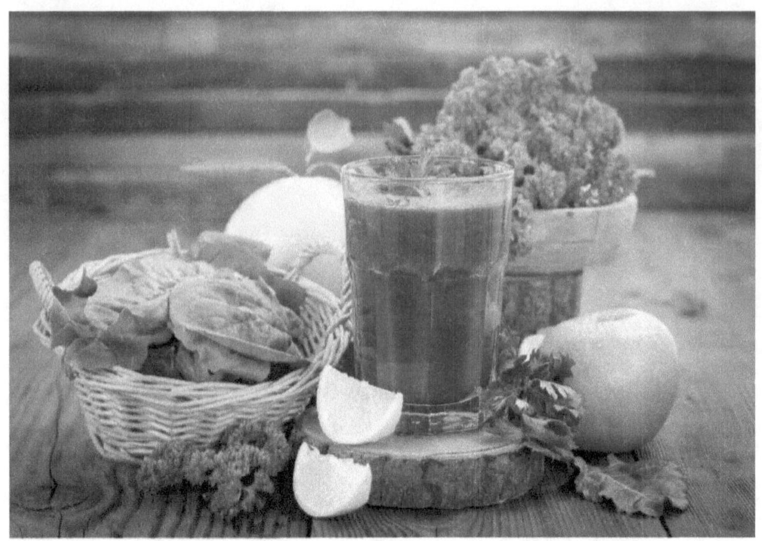

Description: This detox smoothie is a combination of different fruits all of which act as great antioxidants and have lots of vitamin C in them. These fruits improve the metabolic rate of the body and contribute a great deal in reducing the weight.

Preparation Time: 7 minutes.

Serves: 2.

Ingredients:

- Mixed berries, strawberries, raspberries and blueberries- 1 cup
- Apple- 1
- Spinach- 2 cups
- Water or almond milk- 1 cup
- Flax seeds- 1 tablespoon

Directions:

1. Cut and chop the berries of your choice.
2. Peel and slice the apple.
3. Wash, cut and dry the spinach.
4. Take a blender and add in the berries, apple, spinach and the water or almond milk and blend in all the ingredients together.
5. Blend until all the ingredients are mixed properly. You can add more water or almond milk if required.
6. Pour into glasses, top with flax seeds and serve!

Green Protein Detox Smoothie

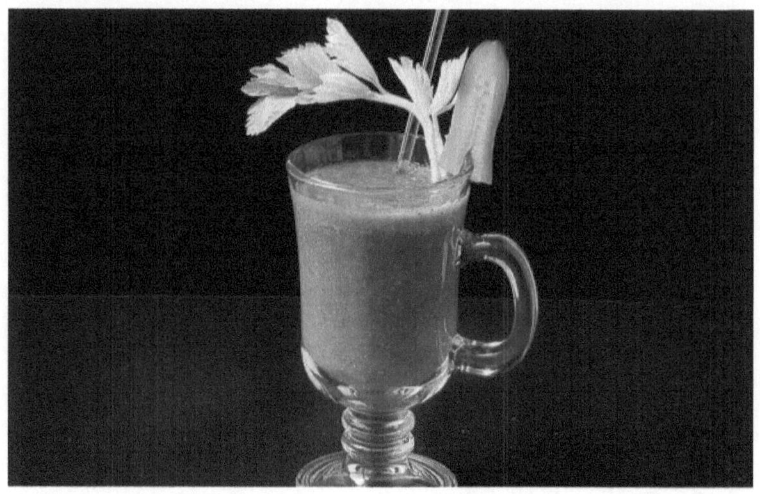

Description: The ideal thing to do is to replace 1 meal a day with these detox green smoothies. These smoothies really contribute a lot to weight loss. These detox smoothies are an excellent way to cleanse your body from all kinds of toxins lying in the body. If you drink these detox smoothies, they will provide you with all kinds of nutrition required by your body.

Ingredients:

- Unsweetened almond milk- ½ cup
- Almond butter- 1 tablespoon
- Banana-1
- Mixed greens for example, spinach, kale etc.- 2 cups

Directions:

1. Cut the banana in small pieces.
2. Wash, dry and cut the greens for example kale, spinach.
3. Take your blender and add in the unsweetened almond milk, almond butter, banana and the greens and blend until all the ingredients are mixed properly.
4. You can add in more almond milk if it is required.
5. Pour into glasses and serve!

Glowing Green Detox Smoothie

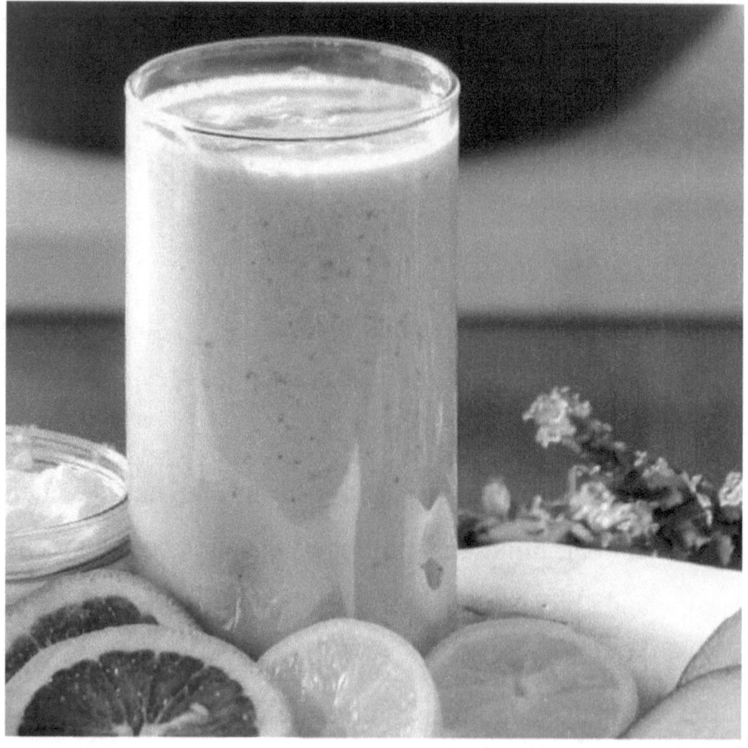

Description: These detox smoothies are not only good for the removal of toxins from your body but they are also a great way to keep your skin young, fresh and healthy. By drinking a glass of smoothie in a day you can have a glowing skin and feel really fresh.

Ingredients:

- Kiwi- 1
- Banana-1
- Pineapple- ¼ cup
- Celery stalks- 2
- Spinach- 2 cups
- Water- 1 cup

Directions:

1. Cut and chop the kiwi.
2. Cut the banana into slices.
3. Cut the pineapple into chunks.
4. Cut and chop the celery stalks.
5. Wash, cut and dry the spinach.
6. Take your nutribullet cup and add in the kiwi, banana, pineapple, celery stalks, spinach and the water and blend.
7. Blend properly to mix all the ingredients.
8. Pour into glasses and serve!

Immortal Elixir

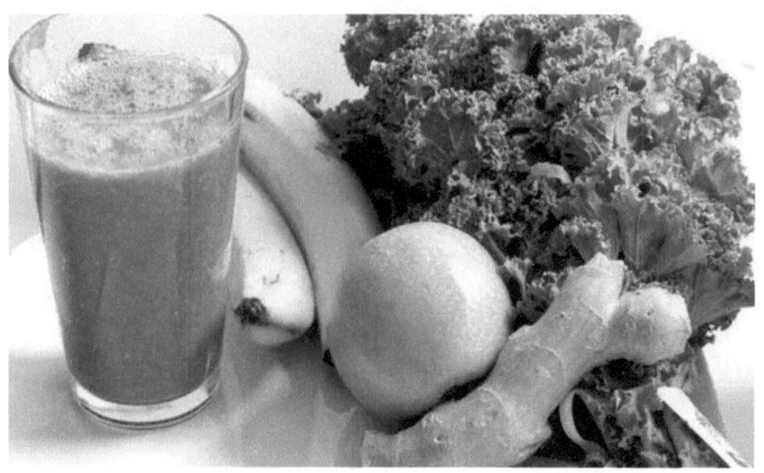

Description: Fruits and vegetables play an important role in the aging process. Some fruits and vegetables are extracted in juice form and made into yummy drinks. Below is the recipe of one such juices.

Preparation Time: 5 minutes

Serves: 2.

Ingredients:

- Parsley- One bunch
- Tomatoes-2
- Kale leaves-2 to 4
- Green apple- 1
- Carrots-1
- Celery stalks-2
- Clove of garlic-1

Directions:

1. In a blender, put in the tomatoes, parsley, kale leaves, green apple, carrots, celery stalks and garlic and water and blend until everything is properly mixed.
2. Pour into glasses and serve chilled.

Wrinkle Beeter

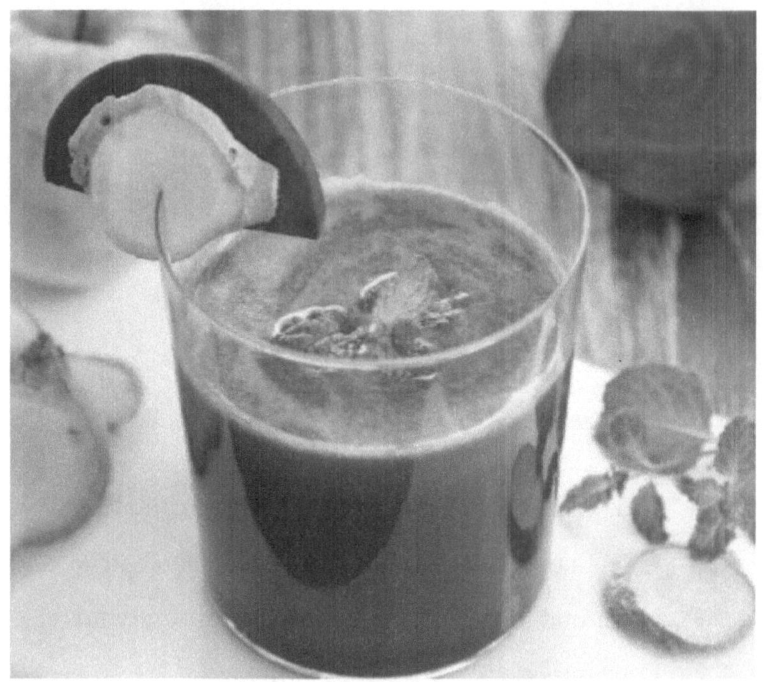

Description: As the name suggests, this drink is for preventing wrinkles from getting formed on the face. This drink is an excellent anti-aging drink and the addition of red beet adds an interesting red color to the drink.

Preparation Time: 5 minutes

Serves: 2.

Ingredients:

- Red beet with stalk-1
- Kale leaves- 4 to 6
- Carrots- 2 to 4
- Apple- 1
- Lemon- half

Directions:

1. In a blender, add in the red beet, kale leaves, carrots, apple and lemon and blend until everything is mixed. Pour into glasses and serve!

Water Melon Detox

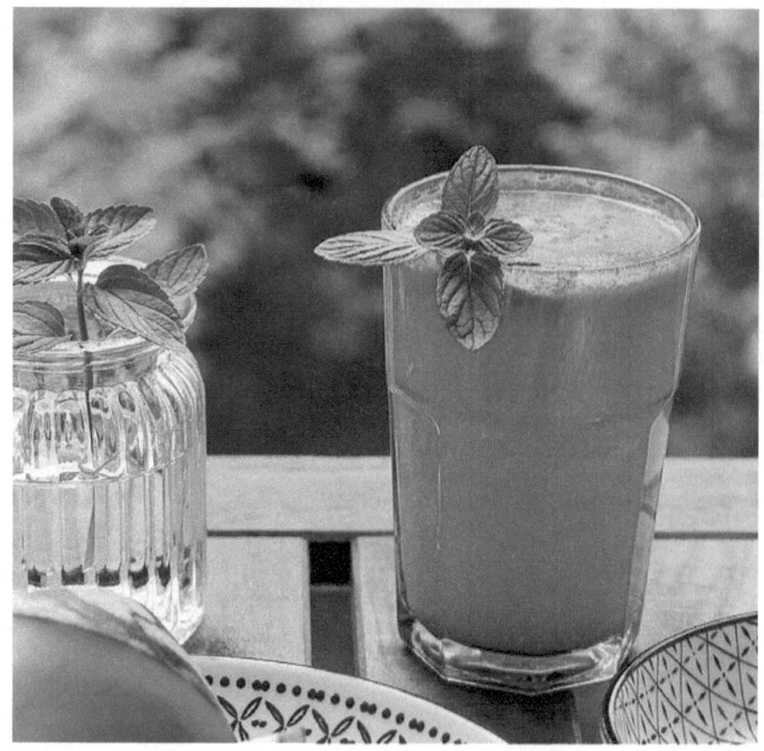

Description: This drink contains water melon which is an excellent anti-aging agent, and it is very good for our bones and for heart health. It has so many vitamins such as vitamin A, C, K.

Preparation Time: 5 minutes

Serves: 2.

Ingredients:

- Watermelon pieces- one cup
- Strawberries- half cup
- Lemon juice-1/4th cup
- Minced ginger-1/4th teaspoon
- Ice -half cup

Directions:

1. In a blender, add in the water melon, strawberries, lemon juice, ginger and the ice. Blend until all the ingredients are mixed properly.
2. Served chilled.

Cucumber Protein Juice

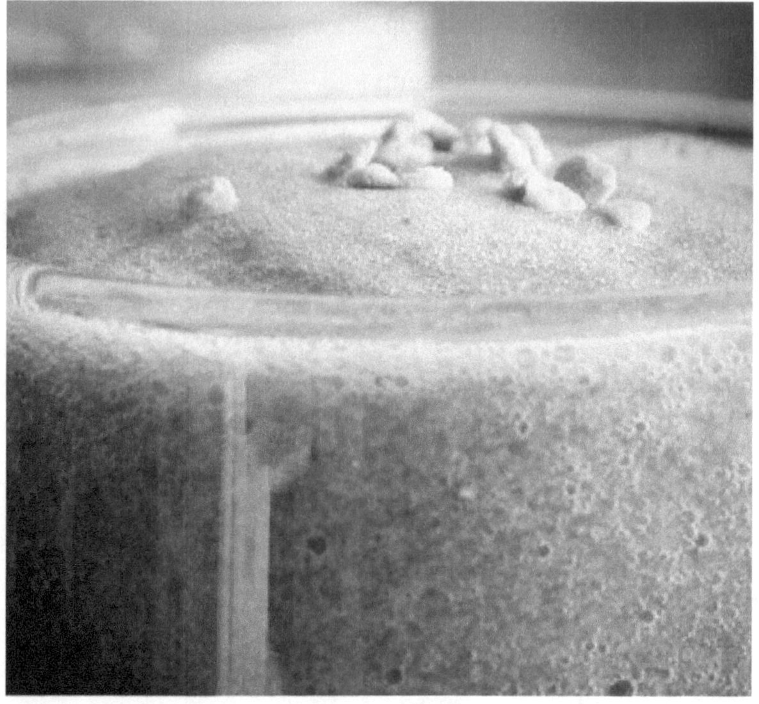

Description: This juice is the perfect anti agent juice, it is good for our complexion, and improves the condition of the hair and nails. It helps in reducing weight and lowers the cholesterol level.

Preparation Time: 8 minutes

Serves: 2.

Ingredients:

- Cucumber- 1
- Apple-1
- Celery stalks-3
- Vanilla protein powder- two teaspoons

Directions:

1. Put the cucumber with the skin in the blender, and add in the apple, celery stalk and the vanilla powder and whisk until all the ingredients are mixed properly.
2. Serve and enjoy!

Spicy Tomato Juice

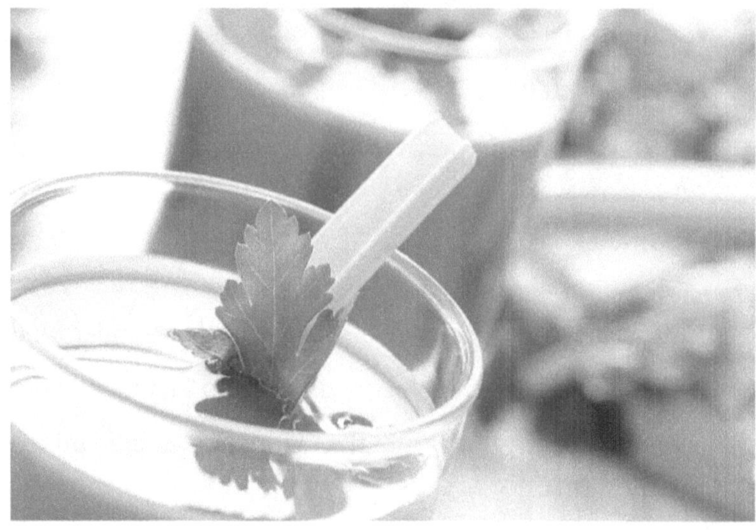

Description: This juice contains a lot of vitamin C and helps prevents lung cancer, prevents heart and lung damage, and reduces the risk of kidney failure and prevents hyper tension. Over all, this juice is one perfect anti aging juice.

Preparation Time: 10 minutes

Serves: 2

Ingredients:

- Ripe tomatoes-3
- Red pepper-half
- Celery stalk-1
- Apple-1
- Yeast- one tablespoon
- Onion powder- Half teaspoon
- Garlic powder- Half teaspoon
- Worcestershire sauce- One teaspoon
- Black pepper- a pinch

Directions:

1. In a blender, add in the tomatoes, bell pepper, celery stalk, apple, yeast, onion powder, garlic powder, the sauce and black pepper and blend until all the ingredients are mixed in properly.
2. Drink this after a heavy exercise or a fast and you will be full and energetic!

Carrot Sunscreen Juice

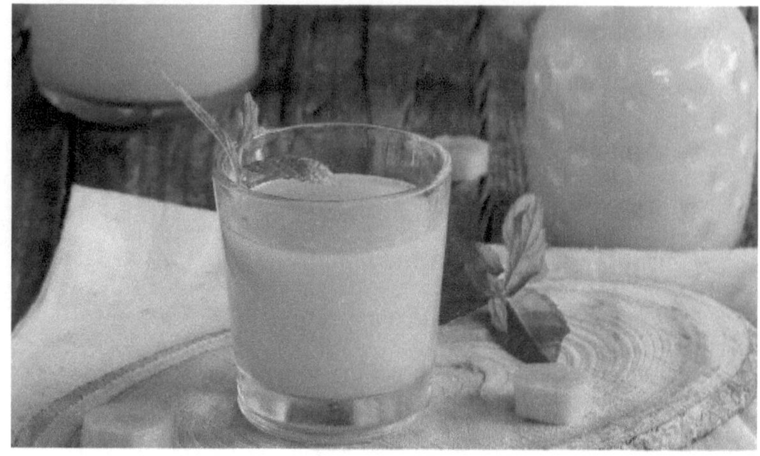

Description: This juice contains both vitamin A and vitamin Cit which reduce the risk of skin cancer, the risk of stroke and reduces the cholesterol levels in the body.

Preparation Time: 5 minutes

Serves: 2.

Ingredients:

- Carrots-6
- celery stalk- 1
- Apple- 1
- Lemon- half

Directions:

1. Put the carrots, celery stalks, apple and lemon in the blender and blend them.
2. Put the lemon with the skin on to get its complete nutrients.
3. Blend and drink when everything is mixed properly.

Virgin Caesar Juice Recipe

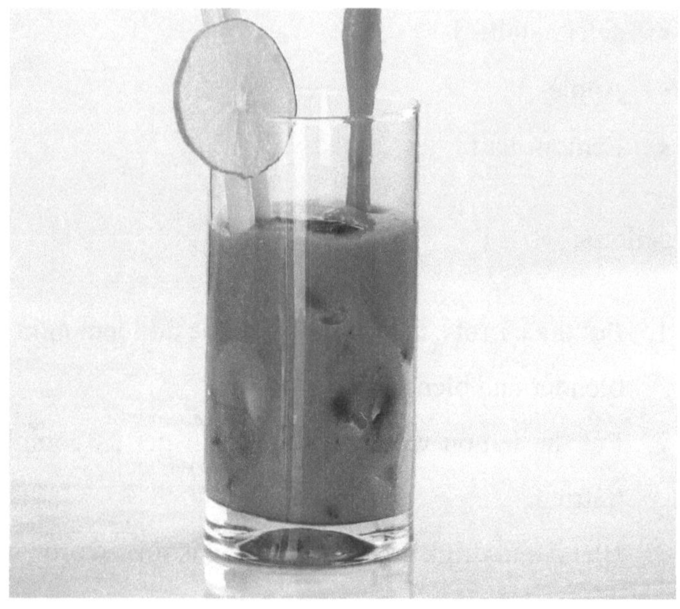

Description: This drink is an excellent anti aging drink in the sense that it prevents lung cancer, reduces the risk of kidney failure and the problem of hyper tension. It also protects the heart from damage and helps prevent smokers.

Preparation Time: 5 minutes

Serves: 2.

Ingredients:

- Tomatoes- 4
- Tabasco sauce- 2 to 5 drops
- Worcestershire sauce- 2 drops
- Celery stalks-2
- Pepper- for taste

Directions:

1. Blend in the tomatoes, Tabasco sauce, Worcestershire sauce, pepper and the celery stalks.
2. Serve the juice chilled.

Tropical Metabolism Booster

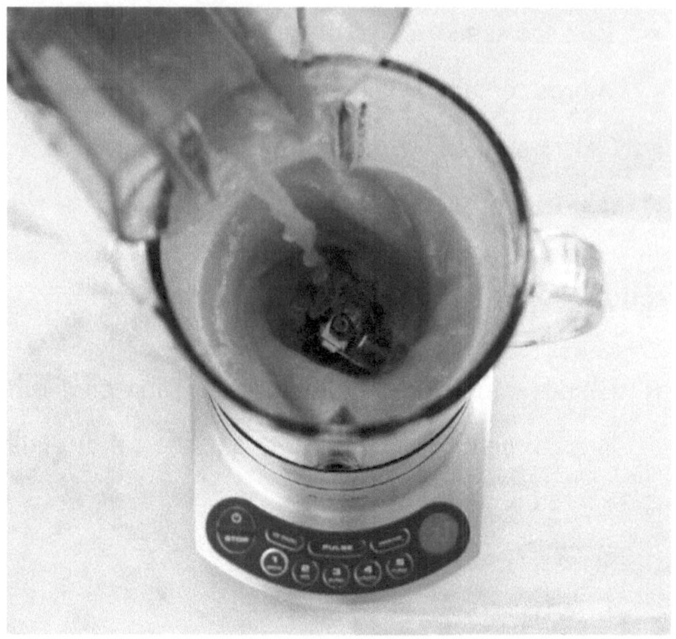

Description: As the name suggests, this drink is for the purpose of speeding up the metabolism process in the human body. The pineapple in this recipe gives the skin a great glow and carrots and cinnamon make the immune system strong.

Preparation Time: 5 minutes

Serves: 2.

Ingredients:

- Pineapple chunks- a few
- Apples-2
- Carrots-2
- Cinnamon-to taste and
- nutmeg to taste

Directions:

1. Add the pineapple, apple, carrots, cinnamon and nutmeg in the blender and blend in all the ingredients properly until mixed.
2. You can serve the drink with ice.

Lemon Juice

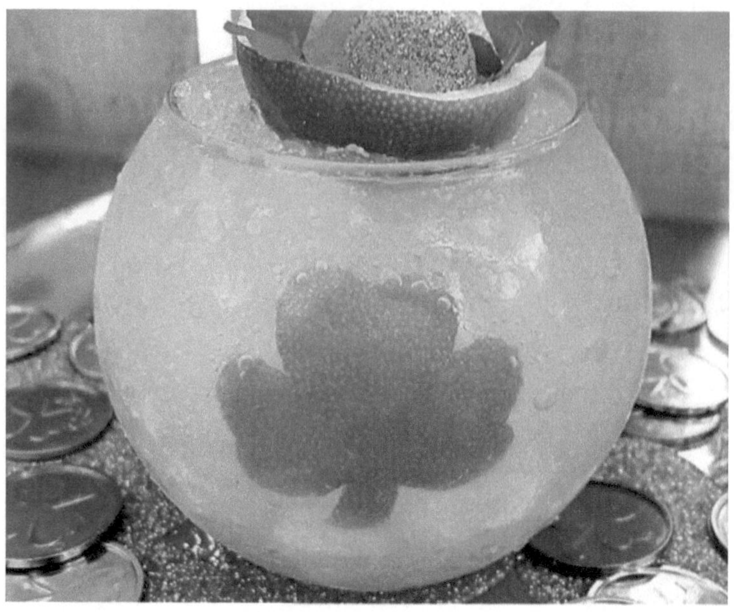

Description: Lemon is a citric fruit. It is very beneficial in a wide variety of ways. The use of lemon in our foods helps prevent cancer from developing. Lemon also gives the skin a very supple, soft and smooth look. Its acidic nature helps fight many bacterias. It is important to include lemon in our diets. One healthy way of including lemon in our diet is by making lemon juice. The following is the recipe of it.

Preparation Time: 5 minutes

Serves: 2 to 4.

Ingredients:

- Lemon- Half kg in season at all times
- Water- 4 glasses
- Ice cubes- as required
- Mint leaves- a few
- Salt- as per taste
- Black pepper- as per your taste
- Sugar- 3 tablespoons

Directions:

1. Take a blender.
2. Take a lemon juicer and squeeze the lemon juice into the blender.
3. Try extracting as much as you can, sieve the seeds aside. Now after the lemon juice, add in the water and now add the ice cubes to make it chilled.
4. Now add the mint leaves, the salt as per your taste, black pepper as per your taste, chop the mint leaves and add in the blender and then add sugar.
5. It is better to use caster sugar as it dissolves much faster.
6. Blend all the ingredients until each of it is mixed properly.
7. Pour the drink into glasses and garnish with more mint leaves.
8. Put in ice cubes and sprinkle with some black pepper if you wish.
9. You can even coat the rims of the glass with either sugar or some lemon juice directly.
10. Enjoy!

DIY Deodorant with Activated Charcoal

Description: Activated charcoal is great for us as it detoxifies the skin and sucks out all kinds of impurities and toxins from the body.

Ingredients:

- Shea butter- 4 ½ tablespoons
- Arrow root powder- 5 tablespoons
- Baking soda- 1 ¼ tablespoons
- Activated charcoal capsules- 2
- Lemon essential oil- 20 drops

Directions:

1. Melt the shea butter on low heat.
2. Once it has melted turn off the heat and then add in the arrow root powder and the baking soda.
3. Now empty the capsules of activated charcoal and add in the mixture.
4. Stir well to form a creamy mixture.
5. Now add in the lemon essential oil and mix it well.
6. Pour this mixture into a glass container and then let it cool for at least 30 minutes before using it.
7. You can even put it in the refrigerator to cool completely before using it.
8. Apply little amounts on your underarms and feel the wonderful fragrance of this deodorant!

Pineapple and Mango Detox Smoothie

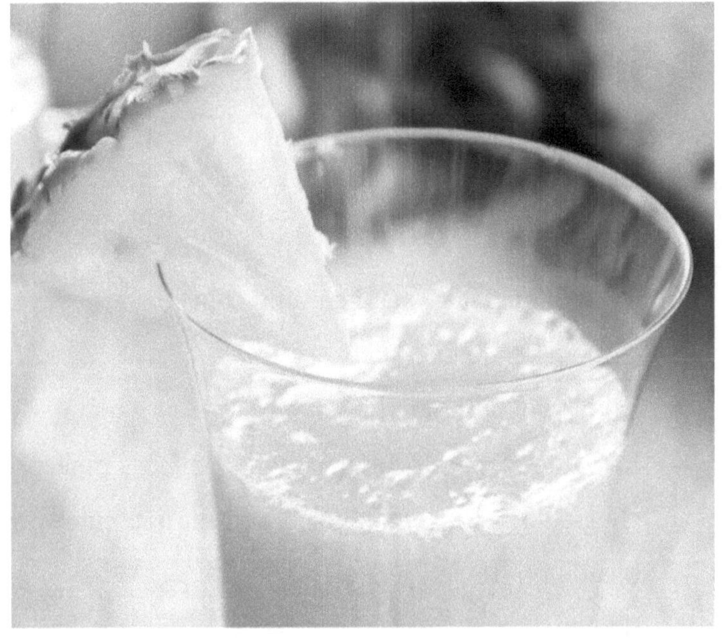

Description: In this smoothie pineapple is added which has great nutritional value. Pineapples are great for the immune system and they are a great citric fruit. The combination of mango and pineapples makes this smoothie very delicious.

Ingredients:

- Ripe mango- 1
- Pineapple - 1
- Yoghurt- 250 grams
- Lemon juice- 1
- Ice cubes- 8

Directions:

1. Take a ripe mango and cut into cubes.
2. Cut pineapple into slices.
3. Whisk yoghurt.
4. In a blender, add in the mango cubes, pineapple slices, yoghurt, lemon juice and the ice cubes and blend until mixed properly.
5. Serve!

Oatmeal

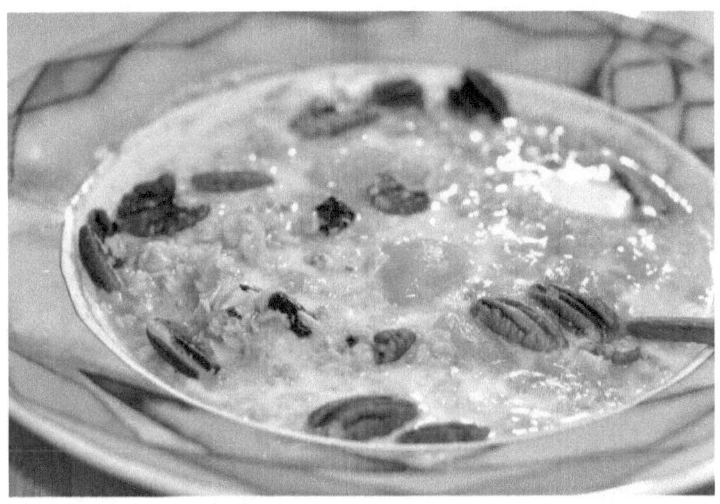

Description: Some foods are anti aging perfect and slow down the process of aging. Oats have low glycemic and contain a lot of nutrients and prevent aging and wrinkles from appearing on the face.

Preparation Time: 5 minutes

Serves: 1.

Ingredients:

- Milk- One bowl
- Quaker oats-2 tablespoons
- Fresh blueberries- around 8 to 10.

Directions:

1. The best way to have oats is in breakfast as porridge.
2. In a bowl, add in the milk, oats and top with blueberries.
3. Any other fruit like strawberry and enjoy the meal.

Orange Custard

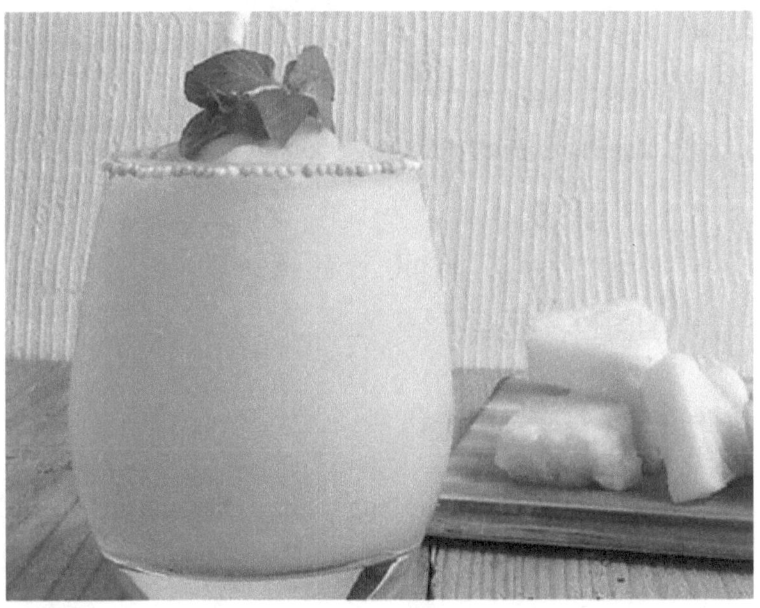

Description: Oranges have a lot of water content in them and are great for the skin. Oranges give the skin and smooth and supple look. Consume the fresh oranges of the season and make a desert with them to avail all the benefits of this fruit.

Preparation Time: 10 minutes

Serves: 6.

Ingredients:

- Eggs- Four
- Egg yolks-2
- Caster sugar-6 oz
- Vanilla extract- One teaspoon
- Milk-16 oz
- Heavy cream-250 ml
- Grated orange zest -1

Directions:

1. In a bowl, beat the eggs, egg yolks, caster sugar, vanilla extract, milk and the cream until all the ingredients are combined.
2. Now add in the orange zest.
3. Grease ramekins and pour the mixture in the ramekins while straining the rind and put in preheated oven to bake on 150 degrees.
4. Bake until they are set.
5. Serve when cool.

Guacamole

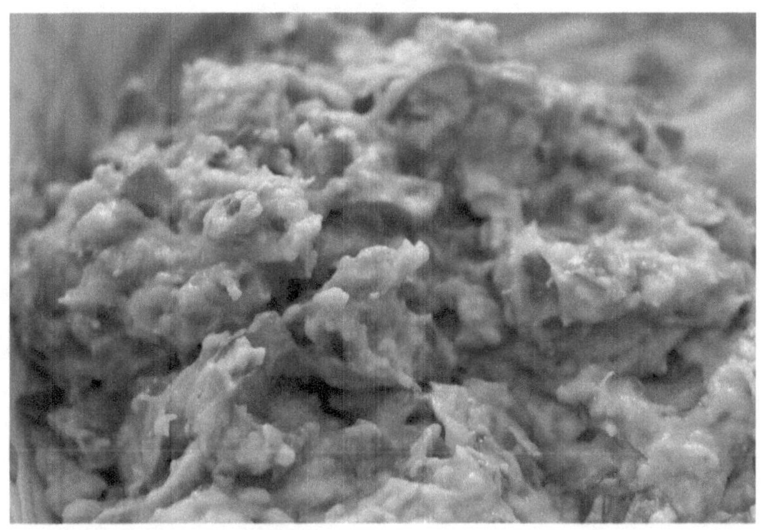

Description: Avocados help to keep the skin hydrated. Avocados also help in absorbing healthy vitamins and nutrients needed by the body. Guacamole is a dish which contains avocados.

Preparation Time: 10 minutes

Makes: 1 cup.

Ingredients:

- Small onion- One
- Small jalapeno- One
- Chopped cilantro-2 tablespoon
- Salt-1/4th teaspoon
- Pepper for taste
- Avocado- One
- Lemon juice- One tablespoon

Directions:

1. In a bowl, add in the onion, jalapeno, cilantro, salt, pepper, lemon juice and avocado.
2. Mash the vegetables with the fork and mix to combine well.
3. Eat it with healthy snacks

Pan Seared Salmon

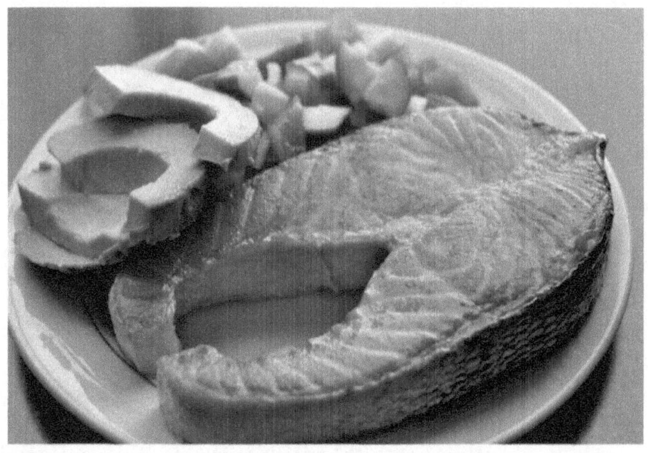

Description: Salmon contains omega 3 which is very beneficial for the skin. Salmon also prevents cancer cells from growing and spreading in the body. Salmon should be consumed twice or thrice in a week.

Preparation Time: 20 minutes

servings: 4

Ingredients:

- Salmon-4 fillets
- Olive oil- Two tablespoons
- Capers- Two tablespoon
- Salt- Pinch
- Black pepper- Pinch
- Lemon-4 slices

Directions:

1. Heat a skillet, coat the salmon fillets with salt, pepper and olive oil and capers.
2. Turn the salmon sides when done on each side.
3. Serve with lemon slices and serve with hot rice.

Green Grape Salad

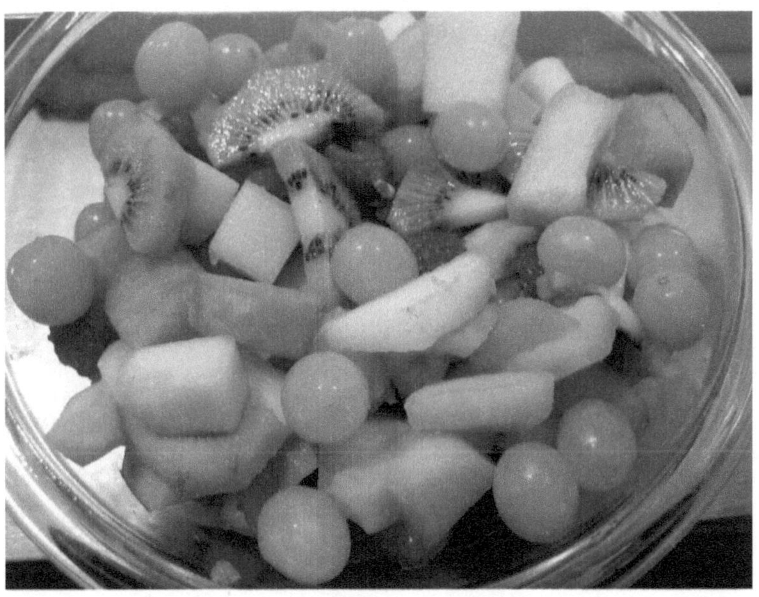

Description: Grapes are known for preventing inflammation in the body. Grapes are also good in keeping the skin glowing and radiant. This hearty green grape salad is perfect as an anti aging recipe.

Preparation Time: 15 minutes

servings: 8

Ingredients:

- Grapes- Four pounds
- Cream cheese- 250 grams
- Sour cream- 250 grams
- White sugar- Half cup
- Vanilla extract- One teaspoon
- Pecans-4 ounces
- Brown sugar-2 tablespoons

Directions:

1. Wash and dry the grapes and in a bowl, add in the cream cheese, sour cream, white sugar, vanilla extract and the grapes until they are coated with the cheese mixture.
2. Sprinkle the pecans and the brown sugar and refrigerate before serving.

Easy Vegetable Beef Soup Recipe

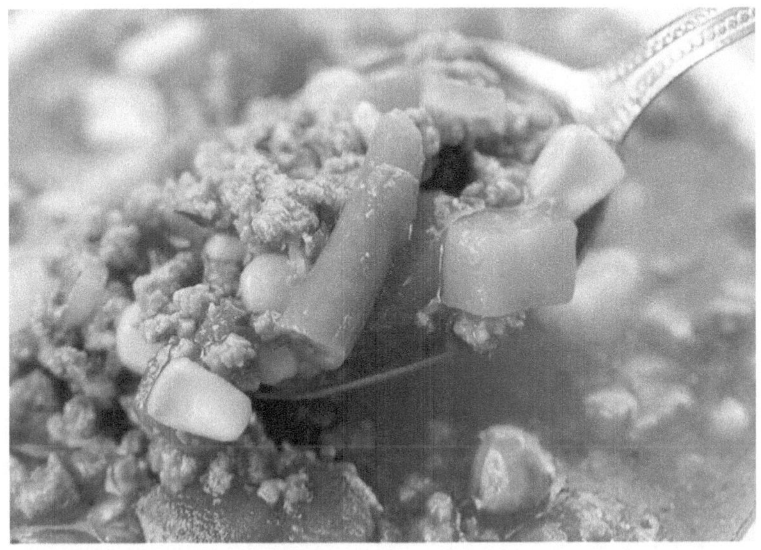

Description: Lean beef is the best way to consume proteins. They are extra ordinarily rich in proteins and make the body's immune system very strong. They also have anti-bacterial properties which help to keep the body strong.

Preparation Time: 3 hours

servings: 16

Ingredients:

- Lean beef-2 pounds
- Mixed vegetables- Four cans
- Tomatoes-4 cans
- Onion- one chopped
- Black pepper- to taste
- Salt- a pinch

Directions:

1. In a pot, cook beef for a few hours until soft and tender.
2. Drain the liquid and now add in the vegetables, tomatoes, onion and let it simmer for 3 to 4 hours.
3. Season with pepper and salt before serving.
4. Serve with prawn crackers.

Roasted Brussel Sprouts

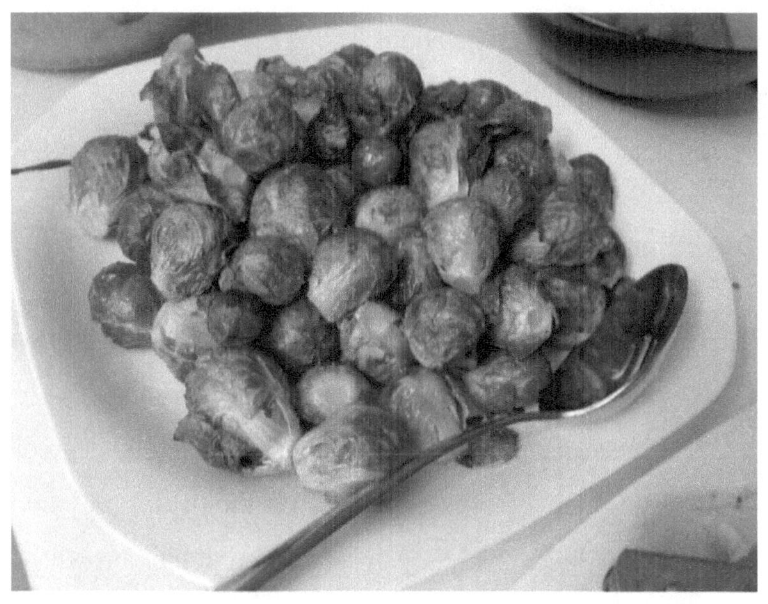

Description: Brussel sprouts have a lot of vitamin A and vitamin C and are a great source of folate. They are exceptionally well for the skin. These roasted brussel sprout are a great and easy dish for your glowing skin.

Preparation Time: 1 hour

Serves: 6.

Ingredients:

- Brussel sprouts- One and half pounds
- Olive oil-3 tablespoons
- Kosher salt- One teaspoon
- Black pepper- Half teaspoon

Directions:

1. Put the brussel sprouts, olive oil, salt and pepper in a plastic bag and coat them with the seasonings.
2. Grease a baking tray and preheat oven to 200 degrees and pour the brussel sprouts on the baking tray and put to bake until they turn nice and golden brown.
3. Turn them halfway if needed.
4. Serve immediately.

Citrus and Kiwi Fruit Salad with Pomegranate and Pistachios

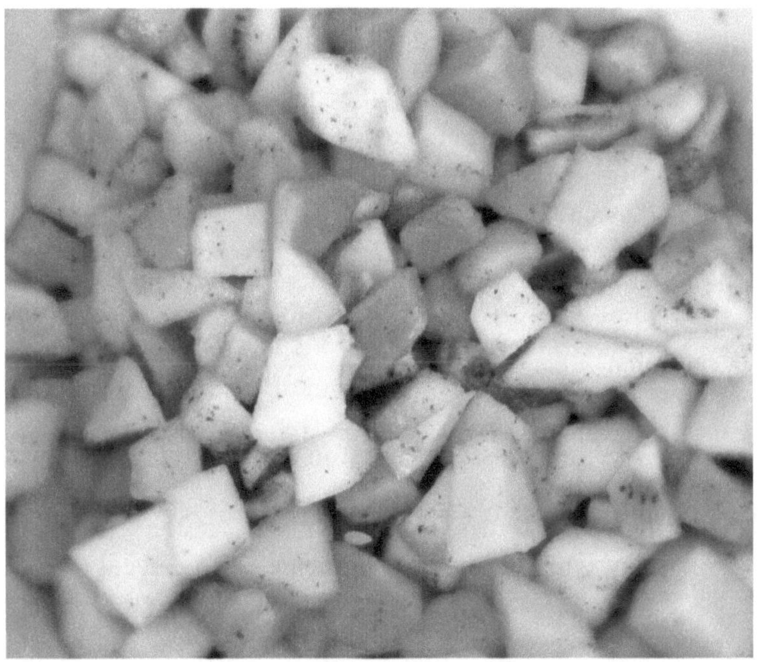

Description: All the citrus fruits such as the oranges, lemons, kiwis are practically loaded with vitamin C. Vitamin c is a very essential component in preventing common cold and flu problems. These fruits also help prevent cancer and cataracs.

Preparation Time: 10 minutes

Serves: 2.

Ingredients:

- Kiwis peeled and sliced- Three
- Oranges peeled and sliced- Four
- Pomegranate seeds-1/4th cup
- Grapefruits sliced-2
- Pistachios chopped- a few
- Orange juice (fresh)- 2 tablespoons optional

Directions:

1. Take few glasses and put in equal amounts of kiwis and oranges in them.
2. Now put in the pomegranate seeds evenly from above.
3. Add in the grapefruits turn by turn now.
4. Drizzle over the orange juice in each glass and in the end, top them with pistachios and serve!

Complete Party Mix with Almonds and Apricots

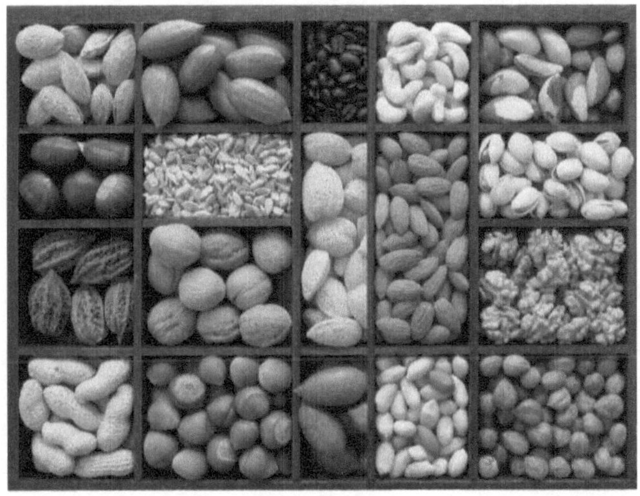

Description: Nuts in particular almonds, pistachios and pine nuts are high in vitamin E. Vitamin E helps a lot in preventing cholesterol level from getting high in the body. A high cholesterol level increases the chances of heart strokes specially with older ages. Nuts are extremely beneficial in keeping the cholesterol level to a balance.

Preparation Time: 30 minutes

Serves: almost 12.

Ingredients:

- Pretzel nuggets- Three cups
- Crispy corn cereal- Three cups
- Almonds- Half cup
- One bag of chips preferably low in sodium
- Chili powder- Two tablespoons
- Cumin- One tablespoon
- Cooking spray
- Salt - One fourth teaspoon
- Dried apricots-half kg

Directions:

1. At first, preheat your oven to 250 degrees.
2. Grease baking tray with butter and add in the pretzel nuggets, the crispy corn cereal, almonds, bag of chips and mix in them the chili powder, cumin, salt and mix well.
3. Roast for a while and then add in the dried apricots and let them bake for another few minutes until all the ingredients are crispy.

Roasted Cauliflower with Capers and Bread Crumbs

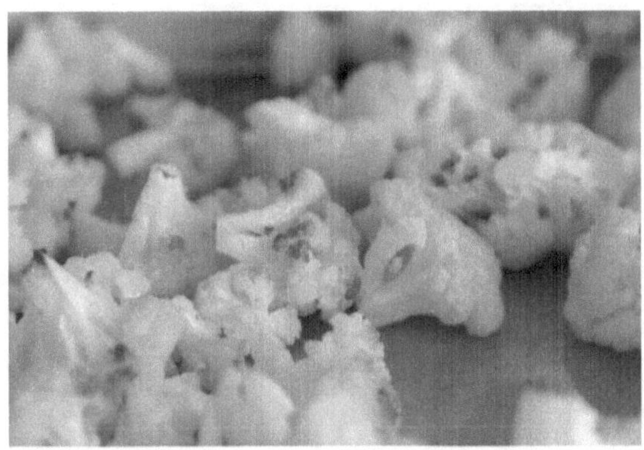

Description: Vegetables such as cauliflower, broccoli, brussel sprouts etc. have a substance in them known as sulforaphane which helps in preventing cancer cells from growing in the body. These vegetables are high in iron and are best in preventing growth of cancer cells.

Preparation Time: 20 minutes

Serves almost 6.

Ingredients:

- Cauliflower-2 heads
- Olive oil- One fourth cup
- Salt- One fourth teaspoon
- Garlic clove peeled-1
- Lemon juice- One fourth cup
- Red chili flakes- One teaspoon
- Drained carpers- Two tablespoons
- Chopped parsley- One fourth cup
- Anchovies fillets-6
- Bread slices-4

Directions:

1. Cut the cauliflower heads and coat them in salt and olive oil and roast in the oven until they turn golden brown for about 20 minutes almost.
2. Toast the bread slices in another separate tray and let them toast.
3. Keep the garlic clove on the bread slices and when cooled and done blend the bread crumbs along with the garlic in a blender to make bread crumbs.
4. In a separate bowl, mash the anchovy fillets and the lemon juice to form a dry paste.
5. Now add in the cauliflower, parsley, carpers, dry chili flakes, bread crumbs and mix.
6. Mix well enough for all ingredients to mix properly.
7. Season with a bit of salt.
8. Serve in bowl!

Strawberry and Banana Green Detox Smoothie

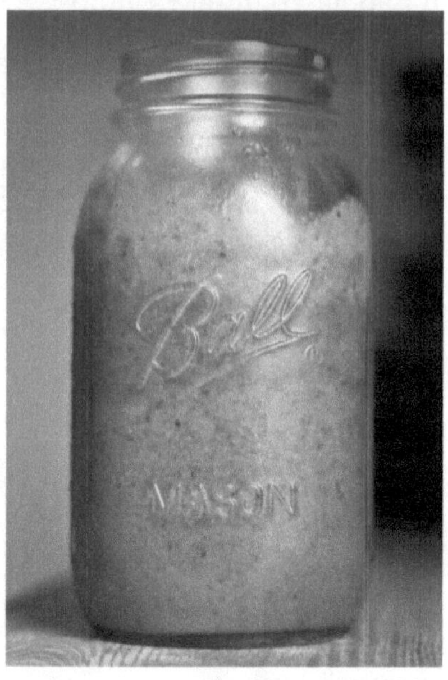

Description: Fruit smoothies are very easy to make, are very nutritious and taste mostly like the fruit. You can hardly taste any of the spinach taste so it is a great option for those who do not like spinach but yet want to take full advantage for their health. Bananas are great antioxidants and contribute to weight loss.

Ingredients:

- Strawberries- ½ cup
- Banana-1
- Spinach- 1 cup
- Almond milk- ½ cup
- Vanilla extract- 1 teaspoon

Directions:

2. Cut the strawberries.
3. Cut the bananas.
4. Wash and cut the spinach.
5. Take your nutribullet cup and add in the strawberries, banana, spinach, almond milk and the vanilla extract and blend.
6. Blend until all the ingredients are mixed properly.
7. Pour and serve!

Conclusion

This book mentions 30 detox recipes which can be extremely beneficial. These 30 detox recipes mention how they can be a great advantage to our skins and our immune systems.

Detox recipes also contribute towards weight loss and keep the skin hydrated. If you wish to be healthy, make your immune system strong and keep your skin healthy and beautiful you need to get the hang of these detox recipes and make them at your home.

We wish you had an amazing time reading this book which consists of 30 amazing detox recipes.

Author's Afterthoughts

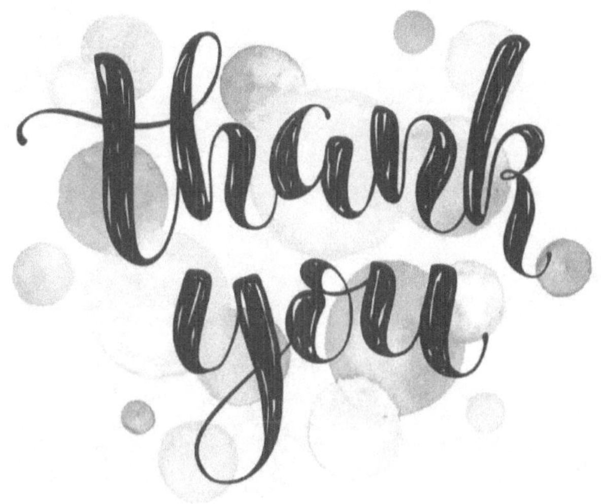

Thanks Ever So Much to Each of My Cherished Readers for Investing the Time to Read This Book!

I know you could have picked from many other books but you chose this one. So, big thanks for buying this book and reading all the way to the end.

If you enjoyed this book or received value from it, I'd like to ask you for a favor. Please take a few minutes to post an honest and heartfelt review on **Amazon.** Your support does make a difference and helps to benefit other people.

Thank you!

Carla Hale

About the Author

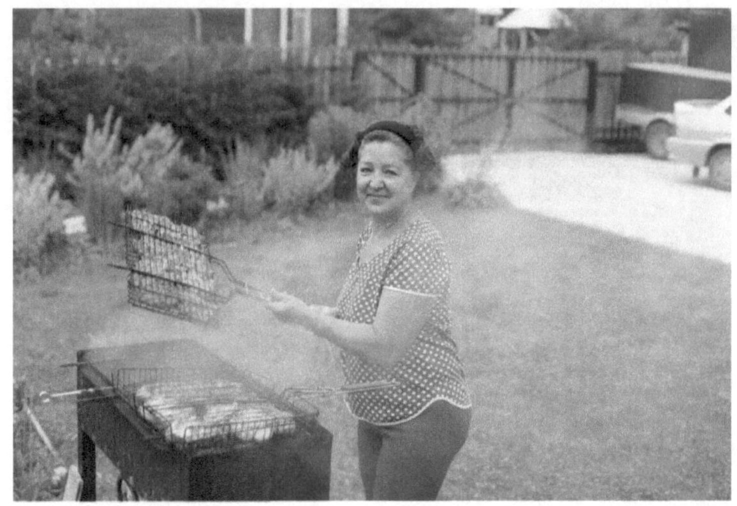

Carla Hale

I think of myself as a foodie. I like to eat, yes. I like to cook even more. I like to prepare meals for my family and friends, I feel like that's what I was born to do…

My name is Carla Hale and as may have suspected already, I am originally from Scotland. I am first and foremost a mother, a wife, but simultaneously over the years I became a proclaimed cook. I have shared my recipes with many and will continue to do so, as long as I can. I like different. I dress different, I love different, I speak different and I cook different. I like to think that I am different because I am more animated about what I do than most; I feel more and care more.

It served me right when cooking to sprinkle some tenderness, love, passion, in every dish I prepare. It does not matter if I am preparing a meal for strangers passing by my cooking booth at the flea market or if I am making my mother's favorite recipe. Each and every meal I prepare from scratch will contain a little bite of my life story and little part of my heart in it. People feel it, taste it and ask for more! Thank you for taking the time to get to know me and hopefully through my recipes you can learn a lot more about my influences and preferences. Who knows you might just find your own favorite within my repertoire! Enjoy!